# Your Free Gift

As a way of saying *thanks* for your purchase, I'm offering a free PDF download of the lab charts included in this book.

With these charts you will be able to take the 63 most important labs with you anywhere you go!

You can download the 4 page PDF document by clicking here, or going to NRSNG.com/labs

# LAB VALUES

## 63 Must Know Labs for Nurses

NursingStudentBooks.com

**Jon Haws RN**

**Sandra Haws RD, CNSC**

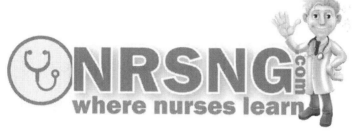

NRSNG.COM | Podcast | YouTube | Facebook | Simclex.com

**If you just want the 4 page PDF of lab values you can find that here.**

## About the Authors

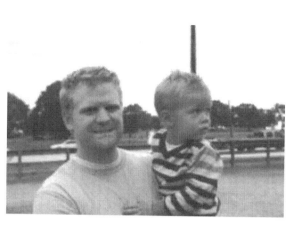

Sick of spending hours and hours trying to find all the information you need for clinical and NCLEX ®study? So was I . . . . That's why I created NRSNG.com, a community of nurses and nursing students wanting to jump start their careers.

I am a registered nurse on a Neurovascular Intensive Care Unit at a Level I Trauma Hospital. I attended college at Brigham Young University and later received my Nursing degree from Methodist College in Peoria, IL. I also hold a Business Management degree from Touro University.

Professionally, I precept nursing students and new graduate Registered Nurses . . . and love it!

Come visit us at NRSNG.com or check in on Facebook.com/NRSNG.

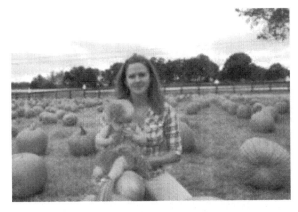

Sandra is a dietitian with one of the largest health care systems in the United States.  She works with intensive care patients.  She obtained her undergraduate degree from Brigham Young University and her graduate degree from Texas Woman's University.  She holds advanced certifications in nutrition support management.

# Table of Contents

# Introduction

Providing comprehensive care for patients requires that all clinicians are competent in the interpretation of laboratory data.

Being able to identify abnormal signs and symptoms in patients, including abnormal diagnostic and laboratory data is required of nurses desiring to provide truly holistic care for their patients.

While the duty of diagnosing and ordering procedures based on data lies on the physician, nurses should verse themselves in lab values, their meanings, normal ranges, and the purpose for each test being ordered.

By understanding lab data and taking the time to assess patient's lab values it becomes possible to participate as part of the interdisciplinary team to affect patient outcomes.

This book is not intended to be used as a means of diagnosing or treating patients and should not take the place of thorough clinical assessment, sound judgment, and institutional guidelines. Normal laboratory data may vary slightly from institution to institution. This book is simply a guide in understanding commonly ordered laboratory data.

This is by no means a comprehensive guide of all available lab tests. There are literally countless clinical tests available to diagnose and treat various conditions. This guide covers some of the most common tests that will be ordered on patients and those tests that should be understood in preparation for passing the boards.

Educating patients on the purpose of tests and the results will lead to greater patient satisfaction and, more importantly will make your patients active participates in their health.  Simple education on the purpose for tests and normal ranges can help ease patients' anxiety and aid them in gaining confidence with the entire medical team.

# Standard Precautions

As with all procedures conducted within the health care setting, it is essential that nurses maintain standard precautions in all patient contact.  Transmission of disease from patient to nurse or between patients can be kept to a minimum through basic adherence to standard precautions.  The CDC outlines the basics behind standard precautions on their website which can be viewed here: http://goo.gl/pVAhtZ.

**Key Components of Standard Precautions:**

- Hand Hygiene
- Proper Use of PPE
- Injection Safety
- Environmental Cleaning
- Medical Equipment
- Respiratory Hygiene

Areas where nurses tend to break standard precautions with patients include the following:

- Not wearing gloves in order to "better feel the vein". Though bare hands increase dexterity it is not worth the risk of transmitting infection.
- Sticking multiple times with one needle. If you fail to obtain a sample with your first stick you must use a new needle.
- Not properly cleaning the area. An alcohol cleansing agent should be used to properly clean the area of injection utilizing the cross hatch method and the area should be allowed to dry prior to needle insertion.
- Not capping needles. Butterfly syringes should be capped immediately upon withdraw from the patient.
- Not properly transferring blood to vacutainers. Blood should only be transferred to containers with shielded transfer devices.

## Order of Blood Draws

Blood collection containers have specific additives to aid in running the tests. It is for this reason that a CBC cannot be placed in the same tube as a BMP for example. In order to prevent cross contamination of additives between tubes it is important that blood is drawn in a very specific order. Upon drawing the sample the vial should be inverted multiple times to insure proper mixing with the additive. For the most up to date information regarding the number of times for inversion please refer to the following website from Quest Diagnostics: http://goo.gl/u7CQ4q .

1. Blood Cultures (including tubes)
2. Light Blue
3. Red/Black
4. Red
5. Green
6. Lavender
7. Royal Blue
8. Gray
9. Yellow

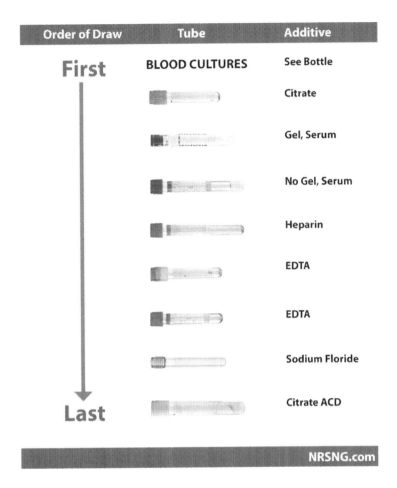

| Order of Draw | Tube | Additive |
|:---:|:---:|:---:|
| **First** | **BLOOD CULTURES** | See Bottle |
| | | Citrate |
| | | Gel, Serum |
| | | No Gel, Serum |
| | | Heparin |
| | | EDTA |
| | | EDTA |
| | | Sodium Floride |
| **Last** | | Citrate ACD |

# Methods of Blood Collection

There are two locations that blood sampling will come from in the adult patient; venous and arterial. The major differences seen on laboratory results will be demonstration in the fact that venous blood is oxygen deficient compared to arterial blood (pH, $CO_2$, $O_2$, Lactic acid). To appropriately assess a patient's respiratory status an arterial sample should be used. Otherwise it is appropriate to use venous or arterial blood (with exceptions for blood cultures) according to institutional guidelines.  In critical care settings many patients will have central lines or arterial lines which provide direct access to blood samples.  When direct access is not possible venous puncture technique can be used to obtain blood samples.

Prior to starting any laboratory draw it is important to pause fluid and TPN infusions (where clinically possible).  Infusions like KPhos, 3%NaCl, and TPN solutions for example can have dramatic effects on laboratory data.  TPN for example can elevate glucose readings up to and above 1000 mg/dL and excessive fluids can dilute venous blood and laboratory readings.

## *Venous Puncture*

When obtaining a sample utilizing venous puncture the following supplies are needed:

1. Tourniquet
2. Butterfly needle
3. Gloves
4. Alcohol
5. Hubs
6. Blood collecting vial
7. Gauze pad
8. Tape

As with all procedures, two forms of patient identification should be provided prior to drawing blood.  Insure that most recent orders have been viewed and maintain aseptic technique while drawing blood. While it can be tempting to aim for the larger veins within the antecubital fossa, patience is needed when searching for a vein that can be palpated with confidence. Depending on how much blood is needed for the sample a smaller distal vein may be used to draw the blood. The goal is to draw from a vein that is palpable.

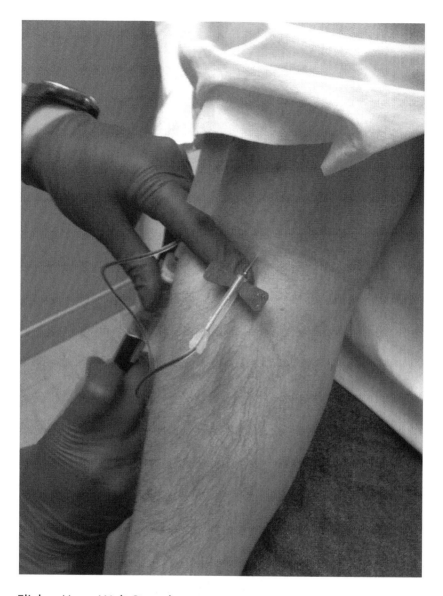

Flicker User: Walt Stoneburner

### Arterial Line Draw

Laboratory samples including, obviously, ABGs can be drawn from arterial lines. With the use of a vamp system there is no need to draw a waste container as the blood drawn back into the vamp serves as the waste. This is helpful for a few reasons; it minimizes the amount of total blood drawn from the patient and can reduce the risk or severity of anemia suffered by patients during hospital stays, and it is slightly faster and easier on the nurse. If blood is being drawn through an art line that does not have a vamp system adequate waste must be drawn prior to drawing labs.

### Central Lines and IVs

Blood sampling can be drawn from existing IVs and central lines utilizing aseptic technique. When drawing from IVs and central lines it is important that proper waste is drawn to avoid a contaminated sample. After blood draws are obtained it is important to flush the line to replace drawn fluid and to insure patent lines.

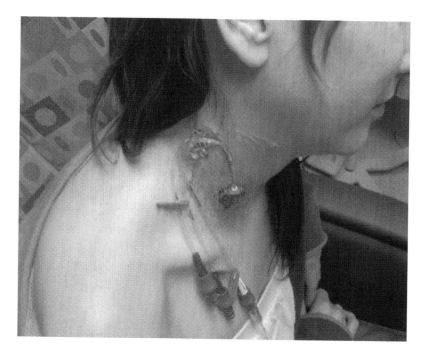

## *Special Considerations*

When drawing any lab it is important to consider additional instructions regarding storage, transportation, and/or drawing technique. Lactic acid for example generally requires being transported to the laboratory on ice, creatinine clearance needs to be collected over 24 hours and refrigerated, blood cultures often have to be taken to the lab by hand. Lab labels, doctors orders, and laboratory orders should be reviewed closely to insure that all special considerations are being considered. Any questions or concerns should be referred to the lab or the ordering doctor.

# Common Laboratory Tests and Values

Again, this is not a complete list of all possible lab tests. These charts include the most common lab values needed to know for the NCLEX®. Studying and knowing these values will prepare you for boards and to provide holistic care for patients.

I created a 4 page PDF download with all these lab values.

## Get a FREE PDF download of these Lab Charts at NRSNG.com/Labs

| Complete Blood Count (CBC) with Differential | | | |
|---|---|---|---|
| **Value** | **Abbreviation** | **Unit** | **Normal Range** |
| Red Blood Cell | RBC | $x10^6$/ml | Male: 4.5 - 5.5 Female: 4.0 - 4.9 |
| White Blood Cell | WBC | cells/mcL | 4,500 - 10,000 |
| Neutrophils | | | 54 - 62% |
| Band Forms | | | 3 - 5% (>8% = left shift) |
| Eosinophlis | | | 1 - 3% |
| Basophils | | | 0 - 0.75% |
| Lymphocytes | | | 25 - 33% |
| Monocytes | | | 3 - 7% |
| Platelets | PLT | cells/mcL | 100,000 - 450,000 |
| Hemoglobin | Hgb | g/dl | Male: 13.5 - 16.5 Female: 12.0 - 15.0 |

| Hematocrit | Hct | % | Male: 41 - 50 Female: 36 - 44 |
|---|---|---|---|
| Mean Corpuscular Volume | MCV | fL | 80 - 100 |
| Red Cell Distribution Width | RDW | | <14.5 |

### Blood Chemistry (Basic Metabolic Panel) (BMP)

| Value | Abbreviation | Unit | Normal Range |
|---|---|---|---|
| Sodium | Na+ | mEq/L | 135 - 145 |
| Potassium | K+ | mEq/L | 3.5 - 5.5 |
| Chloride | Cl- | mEq/L | 96 - 108 |
| Glucose | Glu | mg/dL | 70 - 115 |
| Calcium | $Ca^2+$ | mg/dL | 8.4 - 10.2 |
| Creatinine | Cr | mg/L | 0.7-1.40 |
| Blood Urea Nitrogen | BUN | mg/dL | 7-20 |

### Cholesterol Levels

| Value | Abbreviation | Unit | Normal |
|---|---|---|---|
| Cholesterol Total | | mg/dL | <200 |
| Low Density Lipoprotein | LDL | mg/dL | <70 |
| High Density Lipoprotein | HDL | mg/dL | >60 optimal |
| Triglycerides | | mg/dL | <150 |

## Coagulation Studies

| Value | Abbreviation | Unit | Normal |
|---|---|---|---|
| Prothrombin Time | PT | Seconds | 11 - 14 |
| Partial Thromboplastin Time | PTT | Seconds | 25 - 35 |
| International Normalized Ratio | INR | | 0.8 - 1.2 |
| Activated Partial Thromboplastin Time | aPTT | | 1.5 - 2.5 |

## Arterial Blood Gas

| Value | Abbreviation | Unit | Normal |
|---|---|---|---|
| pH | pH | | 7.35 - 7.45 |
| Partial Pressure of $CO_2$ | $pCO_2$ | mmHg | 35 -45 |
| Partial Pressure of $O_2$ | $pO_2$ | mmHg | 80 - 100 |
| Bicarbonate | $HCO_3$ | mEq/L | 22 - 26 |
| Base Excess | BE | mEq/L | -2 - +2 |
| Oxygen Saturation | $SaO_2$ | % | 95 - 100 |

## Common Laboratory Tests

| Value | Abbreviation | Unit | Normal |
|---|---|---|---|
| Albumin | Alb | g/dL | 3.5 - 6.0 |
| Alkaline Phosphatase | Alk Phos | U/L | 40 - 130 |
| Aspartate Aminotransferase | AST | U/L | 12 - 37 |
| Alanine | ALT | U/L | 13 - 69 |

| | | | |
|---|---|---|---|
| Aminotransferase | | | |
| Activated Partial Thromboplastin Time | aPTT | seconds | 25-39 |
| Ammonia | $NH_3$ | ug/dL | 19 - 60 |
| Amylase | | U/L | 0 - 130 |
| Base Excess (Arterial) | BE | mEq/L | -2 - +2 |
| Bicarbonate (Arterial) | $HCO_3$ | mEq/L | 22 - 26 |
| Bilirubin, Direct (Conjugated) | | mg/dL | 0 - 0.2 |
| Bilirubin, Total | T.billi | mg/dL | 0.1 - 1.2 |
| Blood Urea Nitrogen | BUN | mg/dL | 7-20 |
| Brain Type Natriuretic Peptide | BNP | pg/mL | <100 |
| C-Reactive Protein | CRP | mg/L | <1.0 |
| Calcium | $Ca^2+$ | mg/dL | 8.4 - 10.2 |
| Chloride | Cl- | mEq/L | 96 - 108 |
| Cholesterol Total | | mg/dL | <200 |
| Creatinine | Cr | mg/dL | 0.5 -1.2 |
| Creatinine Clearance | | $mL/min/1.73m^2$ | 85 - 125 |
| Creatine Kinase | CK | U/L | 55 - 170 |
| Creatinine Kinase - MB | CK-MB | ng/mL | <2.40 |
| D-Dimer | DDI | ng/mL | ≤ 250 |
| Erythrocyte Sedimentation Rate | ESR | mm/h | 0 - 20 |
| Ferritin | | ng/mL | 20-300 |

| | | | |
|---|---|---|---|
| Folic Acid | | ng/mL | 2 - 20 |
| Glomerular Filtration Rate | GFR | mL/min/1.73 m2 | 60 |
| Glucose | Glu | mg/dL | 70 - 115 |
| Glucose Tolerance Test | GTT | mg/dL | Fasting: 60-100 1 hour: <200 2 hours: < 140 |
| Glycosolated Hemoglobin | HgbA1c | % of total Hgb | 5.6-7.5 |
| Growth Hormone | GH | ng/mL | Male: <5 Female: < 10 |
| Hematocrit | Hct | % | Male: 41 - 50 Female: 36 - 44 |
| Hemoglobin | Hgb | g/dl | Male: 13.5 - 16.5 Female: 12.0 - 15.0 |
| High Density Lipoprotein | HDL | mg/dL | >60 optimal |
| Homocysteine | | mg/L | 0.54 - 2.3 |
| International Normalized Ratio | INR | | 0.8 - 1.2 |
| Iron | Fe | ug/dL | 50-175 |
| Lactate Dehydrogenase | LDH | U/L | 88-230 |
| Lactic Acid | | mEq/L | Venous |

| | | | Blood: 0.5-2.2 Arterial Blood: 0.5-1.6 |
|---|---|---|---|
| Lipase | | U/L | 23 - 300 |
| Low Density Lipoprotein | LDL | mg/dL | <70 |
| Magnesium | Mg | mg/dL | 1.6 – 2.6 |
| Mean Corpuscular Volume | MCV | fL | 80 - 100 |
| Myoglobin | MB | ng/mL | 5 – 70 |
| Osmolality, Serum | | mOSM/kg | 261-280 |
| Oxygen Saturation (Arterial) | $SaO_2$ | % | 95 - 100 |
| Partial Pressure of (Arterial) $CO_2$ | $pCO_2$ | mmHg | 35 -40 |
| Partial Pressure of (Arterial) $O_2$ | $pO_2$ | mmHg | 80 - 100 |
| Partial Thromboplastin Time | PTT | Seconds | 25 - 35 |
| pH (arterial) | pH | | 7.35 - 7.45 |
| Phosphorus (phosphate) | $PO_4$ | mg/dL | 3.0-4.5 |
| Platelets | PLT | cells/mcL | 100,000 - 450,000 |
| Potassium | K+ | mEq/L | 3.5 - 5.5 |
| Prealbumin | PAB | mg/dL | 19-38 |
| Prostate Specific | PSA | ng/mL | Male: < |

| | | | |
|---|---|---|---|
| Antigen | | | 4<br>Female:<br>< 0.5 |
| Protein (total) | Prot | g/dL | 6-8 |
| Prothrombin Time | PT | Seconds | 11 - 14 |
| Red Blood Cell | RBC | $x10^6$/cells/mm$^3$ | Male:<br>4.5 - 5.5<br>Female:<br>4.0 - 4.9 |
| Red Cell Distribution Width | RDW | | <14.5 |
| Sodium | Na+ | mEq/L | 135 - 145 |
| Triglycerides | TG | mg/dL | <150 |
| Total Iron Binding Capacity | TIBC | ug/dL | 250-460 |
| Troponin I | cTnI | ng/mL | <0.035 |
| White Blood Cell | WBC | cells/mcL | 4,500 - 10,000 |

# Get a FREE PDF download of these Lab Charts at NRSNG.com/Labs

# Explanation of Lab Values

# Albumin

## Normal

3.5 - 6.0 g/dL

## Indications

evaluation of chronic illness, liver disease, or nutritional status

## Description

Albumin is a transport protein in the blood. It helps maintain the oncotic pressure of the blood. Albumin levels will drop if synthesis is slowed, protein intake is inadequate, or there are increased losses. Albumin has a long half life, however, so levels are not a good indicator of acute illness.

## What would cause increased levels?

dehydration, hyper infusion of albumin

## What would cause decreased levels?

inadequate intake, liver disease, inflammation, chronic disease, losses (fistula, hemorrhage, kidney disease, burns), over hydration, Increased catabolism, congestive heart failure

# Alkaline Phosphatase

## Normal

40-130 U/L

## Indications

identifying hepatobiliary disease, malignancies, bone disease, bone damage in renal patients; useful in evaluating bone growth in children.

## Description

Alkaline phosphatase (ALP) is located in several places in the body: liver, intestines, biliary tract, bones, placenta. Different isoenzymes of ALP can be used to determine different disorders: liver, bone, intestine, certain cancers. It can also be used to determine bone turnover in postmenopausal women.

## What would cause increased levels?

liver disease, bone disease, pregnancy, amyloidosis, lung cancer, pancreatic cancer, congestive heart failure, ulcerative colitis, Hodgkin's disease, chronic renal failure, sarcoidosis

## What would cause decreased levels?

hypophophatasia, anemia, kwashiorkor, cretinism, hypothyroidism, zinc or magnesium deficiency, scurvy

# Aspartate Aminotransferase

## Normal

12-37 U/L

## Indications

monitor progression of liver disease, and response to treatments.

## Description

Aspartate aminotranferase (AST) is an enzyme primarily found in liver and heart cells. To a smaller extent it is also found in pancreas, kidneys, skeletal muscle, and brain.

## What would cause increased levels?

Liver disease, shock, pancreatitis, CHF, Liver Cancer, dermatomyositis, muscular dystrophy, biliary tract obstruction

## What would cause decreased levels?

CVA, delirium tremens, pericarditis, cirrhosis, hemolytic anemia

# Alanine Aminotransferase

### Normal

13 – 69 U/L

### Indications

monitoring progression of liver disease or liver damage. It can also aid in monitoring response to treatments

### Description

ALT is an enzyme made in the liver. This enzyme is found in highest concentrations in the liver, but is found to lesser extent in heart, skeletal muscle and kidney. Damage to the liver results in a significant increase in this enzyme.

### What would cause increased levels?

cirrhosis, muscle damage, preeclampsia, biliary tract obstruction, burns, Pancreatitis, long-term alcohol abuse, Liver Cancer, muscular dystrophy, MI, myositis, shock, infections mononucleosis

### What would cause decreased levels?

pyridoxal phosphate deficiency

# Activated Partial Thromboplastin Time

## Normal

25-39 seconds

## Indications

identifying congenital deficiencies in clotting; monitoring effects of liver disease, protein deficiency, fat malabsorption on clotting.

## Description

APPT is a test that measures the amount of time it takes for a fibrin clot to form after reagents have been added to the specimen. It is useful in diagnosis clotting disorders. In conjunction with PT it can be used to differentiate the specific factor that may be missing.

## What would cause increased levels?

vitamin K deficiency, DIC, patients on hemodialysis, afibrinogenemia, polycythemia, liver disease, Von Willebrand disease.

## What would cause decreased levels?

N/A

# Ammonia

### Normal

19-60 µg/dL

### Indications

identifying liver disease, monitoring hepatic encephalopathy, and evaluating effectiveness of treatment.

### Description

Ammonia is a byproduct created when protein is broken down. Ammonia is converted into urea in the liver, and urea is excreted by the kidneys. During liver disease ammonia levels rise and can have a negative effect on the brain.

### What would cause increased levels?

gastrointestinal hemorrhage, liver failure, hepatic coma, Reye's syndrome, TPN

### What would cause decreased levels?

N/A

# Amylase

**Normal**

0-130 U/L

**Indications**

diagnosing pancreatitis, macroamylasemia, pancreatic duct obstruction, trauma to pancreas.

**Description**

Amylase is made in the pancreas. It is an enzyme that breaks down carbohydrate to allow our body to absorb it. Monitoring amylase levels can identify problems with the pancreas

**What would cause increased levels?**

alcoholism, pancreatitis, DKA, peritonitis, abdominal trauma, pancreatic cancer, duodenal obstruction, gastric resection, mumps, pancreatic cyst

**What would cause decreased levels?**

cystic fibrosis, liver disease, pancreatic insufficiency, pancreatectomy

# Base Excess

## Normal

-2 - +2 mEq/L

## Indications

identifying metabolic acidosis and alkalosis

## Description

Base excess represents the amount of anions in the blood that can help buffer against changes in pH. Base excess is altered when bicarbonate levels are either high or low. If base excess is low or high it indicates a metabolic cause of acidosis or alkalosis. Negative base excess indicates metabolic acidosis.

## What would cause increased levels?

metabolic alkalosis (alkali ingestion, gastric suctioning, low potassium, Cushing's disease, diuresis, diarrhea, vomiting)

## What would cause decreased levels?

Metabolic acidosis (DKA, Addison's disease, Wilson's disease, renal failure, diarrhea, fistula, increased acid intake)

# Bicarbonate

## Normal

22-26 mEq

## Indications

differentiate between metabolic and respiratory causes of pH imbalances.

## Description

Bicarbonate is a base and anion that helps to neutralize acids in the blood.  Bicarbonate needs to be 20 times carbonic acid to maintain balance in the blood.  Bicarbonate $HCO_3^-$ levels can either be measured or determined using carbon dioxide levels

## What would cause increased levels?

anoxia, respiratory acidosis, metabolic alkalosis

## What would cause decreased levels?

hypocapnia, respiratory alkalosis, metabolic acidosis

# Direct Bilirubin

### Normal

0-0.2 mg/dL

### Indications

useful when used in correlation with total bilirubin, used to determine amount of unconjugated bilirubin, an elevated unconjugated bilirubin indicates a problem with the liver

### Description

Bilirubin is a byproduct of red blood cell breakdown. Bilirubin is transported to the liver where it is conjugated. It then goes to the intestines to be excreted. Direct bilirubin is a measure of conjugated bilirubin. If you subtract direct bilirubin from total bilirubin you can determine the amount of unconjugated bilirubin. If unconjugated bilirubin is elevated that is specific to liver disease

### What would cause increased levels?

elevated destruction of red blood cells, liver problems

### What would cause decreased levels?

N/A

# Total Bilirubin

## Normal

0.1 - 1.2 mg/dL

## Indications

identifying liver disease, obstructive jaundice, biliary disease, newborn jaundice, and effectiveness of treatment.

## Description

One of the by-products of red blood cell breakdown is bilirubin. Bilirubin is made in the bone marrow, liver, or spleen and is transported by albumin to the liver. In the liver bilirubin is conjugated. In the small intestine conjugated bilirubin is eventually excreted in the feces as urobilin. Excess bilirubin causes a yellowing of the skin and the whites of the eyes called jaundice.

## What would cause increased levels?

post-blood transfusions, hematoma, newborn jaundice, pernicious anemia, hepatic jaundice, liver tumors, biliary obstruction, Gilbert's disease, alcoholism, cholesytitis, cholangitis, cirrhosis, hepatitis, Mono, hypothyroidism, breast milk jaundice.

## What would cause decreased levels?

N/A

# Blood Urea Nitrogen

### Normal

7-20 mg/dL

### Indications

identify liver problems, renal problems, hydration status, tumor lysis; evaluate effects of drugs on liver or kidney; monitor effectiveness of hemodialysis

### Description

When protein is broken down ammonia is formed. Ammonia is converted to urea in the liver and is eventually excreted in the kidneys. Blood urea nitrogen (BUN) measures the amount of urea in the blood.

### What would cause increased levels?

renal failure, CHF, kidney disease, DM, excessive protein intake, GI bleed, shock, dehydration, ketoacidosis, neoplasm, urinary tract obstruction.

### What would cause decreased levels?

liver failure, over-hydration, inadequate protein intake, pregnancy

# Brain Type Natriuretic Peptide

## Normal

<100 pg/mL

## Indications

identify congestive heart failure, effectiveness of treatment, or severity of disease.

## Description

Brain natriuretic peptide (BNP) is a hormone.  It is made by the heart and indicates how hard the heart is working.  When levels are increased  it indicates that the heart is working too hard

## What would cause increased levels?

CHF

## What would cause decreased levels?

N/A

# C-Reactive Protein

## Normal

<1.0 mg/L

## Indications

differentiate between appendicitis vs pelvic inflammatory disease, Crohn's vs ulcerative colitis, rheumatoid arthritis and lupus (SLE - systemic lupus erythematosus); monitor or identify inflammation in the body, evaluate coronary artery disease.

## Description

C-reactive protein (CRP) is made in the liver in response to inflammation. CRP helps practitioners identify inflammation and when it has resolved. CRP is a good indicator because it increases quickly in the inflammatory response, and drops when inflammation resolves.

## What would cause increased levels?

bacterial infection, Crohn's disease, inflammatory bowel disease, lupus, rheumatoid arthritis, pregnancy, myocardial infarction.

## What would cause decreased levels?

N/A

# Calcium

## Normal

8.4-10.2 mg/dL

## Indications

identify problems with parathyroid, diseases that affect bone, effectiveness of treatments.

## Description

Calcium ($Ca^+$) is a positive ion in the body. The parathyroid gland and Vitamin D are responsible for Calcium regulation in the body. Calcium is primarily located in bone and teeth, but is also found in the blood and inside cells. Other than a major component of bone, Calcium also participates in muscle contraction. In the blood about 45% of Calcium travels in ion form, 40% is bound to proteins like albumin, 15% bound to anions like bicarbonate, lactate, etc. When albumin levels are low, Calcium levels will appear lower. Calcium has an important relationship with Phosphorus: they are inversely proportional.

## What would cause increased levels?

cancers (lymphoma, leukemia, bone), acidosis, dehydration, excess Ca intake, hyperparathyroidism, pheochromocytoma, polycythemia vera, renal transplant, sarcoidosis, vitamin D toxicity.

## What would cause decreased levels?

malnutrition, cirrhosis, hypoparathyroidism, alkalosis, chronic renal failure, Magnesium deficiency, hypoalbunemia, hyperphosphatemia, malabsorption, alcoholism, osteomalacia, Vitamin D deficiency.

# Chloride

## Normal

97-107 mEq/L

## Indications

identify different types of acidosis.

## Description

Chloride (Cl⁻) is an anion found in the blood. Sodium and chloride help maintain oncotic pressure and water balance in the body. Chloride is inversely related to bicarbonate levels in the blood. Chloride is a part of HCL which is utilized in the stomach to breakdown food. When red blood cells take up $CO_2$ they take up chloride as well. The negative ion bicarbonate then leaves the red blood cell so that the electrical charge is maintained. Extra chloride is excreted into the urine by the kidneys.

## What would cause increased levels?

dehydration, acute renal failure, Cushing's disease, hyperparathyroidism, metabolic acidosis, respiratory alkalosis.

## What would cause decreased levels?

congestive heart failure, overhydration, water intoxication, burns, metabolic alkalosis, Addison's disease, salt-losing nephritis, excessive sweating, diarrhea, vomiting, fistula.

# Cholesterol

## Normal

<200 mg/dL

## Indications

determine risk of cardiovascular disease; diagnose nephrotic disease, hepatic disease, pancreatitis; gauge response to treatment.

## Description

Cholesterol (Chol) is a lipid in the body. It is a part of cell membranes, a precursor for vitamin D, steroids, bile acids. Cholesterol is primarily synthesized in the liver and intestines. It is transported via lipoproteins. There are multiple types of lipoproteins and they each have slightly different functions: high-density lipoprotein (HDL), low-density lipoprotein, LDL, very low-density lipoprotein (VLDL).

## What would cause increased levels?

tangier disease, myeloma, burns, pernicious anemia, thalassemia, waldensrom's macroglobulinemia, chronic myelocytic leukemia, malabsorbtion, malnutrition, liver disease, polycythemia vera, chronic obstructive pulmonary disease, hyperthyroidism, myeloma

## What would cause decreased levels?

Gout, Obesity, high fat diet, pregnancy, nephrotic syndrome, werner's syndrome, von Gierke disease, alcoholism, anorexia, ischemic heart disease, acute intermittent porphyria, pancreatic malignancy

# Creatinine

**Normal**

0.5-1.2 mg/dL

**Indications**

identify muscular disorders or renal disease.

**Description**

Creatinine is a byproduct of creatine metabolism, and it is excreted in the kidneys. Creatinine is created in proportion to muscle mass and usually stays stable.

**What would cause increased levels?**

gigantism, dehydration, shock, renal disease, rhabdomyolysis, acromegaly, CHF, hyperparathyroidism

**What would cause decreased levels?**

loss of muscle mass, inadequate protein intake, pregnancy, liver disease, muscular dystrophy

# Creatinine Clearance

### Normal

Male: 97 to 137 ml/min
Female: 88 to 128 ml/min

### Indications

used to determine kidney damage in renal disease, glomerular function, effectiveness of treatment.

### Description

Creatinine is a byproduct of creatine metabolism, and it is excreted in the kidneys. Creatinine is created in proportion to muscle mass and usually stays stable. Urine and blood levels are compared to determine creatinine clearance from the blood.

### What would cause increased levels?

DM, exercise, renal disease, tuberculosis, acromegaly, gigantism, congestive heart failure, high protein diet, polycystic kidney disease, dehydration, infections, hypothyroidism.

### What would cause decreased levels?

glomerulonephritis, paralysis, vegetarian diet, anemia, leukemia, shock, muscle wasting, hyperparathyroidism, polycystic kidney disease

# Creatine Kinase

## Normal

55 - 170 U/L

## Indications

diagnose acute MI, ischemia, dermatomyosis, muscular dystrophy; evaluate success of treatment

## Description

Creatine Kinase enzyme is found in heart and skeletal muscle and to a lesser extent brain. When damage is done to these types of tissue CK is released into the blood. There are three isoenzymes, and depending on which one is elevated this lab value can help one determine timing, location, extent of damage. The three isoenzymes are CK-MB (cardiac), CK-MM (skeletal), and CK-BB (brain).

## What would cause increased levels?

alcoholism, brain infarction, congestive heart failure, delirium tremens, dermatomyositis, head injury hypothyroidism, hypoxic shock, infectious disease, gastrointestinal tract infection, loss of blood supply to muscle, muscular dystrophy, myocardial infarction, myocarditis, neoplasms of the prostate, bladder of GI tract, polymyositis, pregnancy, hypothermia, pulmonary edema, pulmonary embolism, reye's sydrome, rhabdomyolysis, surgery, tachycardia, tetanus, trauma.

## What would cause decreased levels?

small stature, sedentary lifestyle

# Creatine Kinase -MB

### Normal

< 2.40 ng/mL

### Indications

diagnose acute MI, identify ischemia

### Description

Creatine Kinase enzyme is found in heart and skeletal muscle and to a lesser extent brain. When damage is done to these types of tissue CK is released into the blood. There are three isoenzymes, and depending on which one is elevated this lab value can help one determine timing, location, extent of damage. The three isoenzymes are CK-MB (cardiac), CK-MM (skeletal), and CK-BB (brain). If CK-MB is elevated 3 times more than CK this indicates damage to heart muscle

### What would cause increased levels?

damage to the heart including ischemia, surgery, trauma, inflammation; kidney failure

### What would cause decreased levels?

n/a

# D-Dimer

**Normal**

≤ 250 ng/mL

**Indications**

Identify DIC and rule out pulmonary embolism, DVT, or stroke.

**Description**

D-dimer is a compound formed when two identical fibrin molecules combine. Cross-linkages do not occur between fibrinogen molecules. D-dimer levels are elevated in the setting of clot breakdown, but will be even higher in the setting of DIC

**What would cause increased levels?**

surgery, trauma, infection, liver disease, cancer, pregnancy, DVT, DIC, cardiac disease

**What would cause decreased levels?**

N/A

# Erythrocyte Sedimentation Rate

**Normal**

0-20 mm/h

**Indications**

identifies inflammation which assists in diagnosing cancer, infection, and autoimmune diseases.

**Description**

The erythrocyte sedimentation rate (ESR) test measures sedimentation of red blood cells. The inflammatory process affects proteins in the blood which causes red blood cells to stick together and settle out of liquid. Normal blood has very little settling, but during the inflammatory process the ESR is elevated.

**What would cause increased levels?**

myocardial infarction, anemia, cancers, systemic lupus erythromatosus, Crohn's disease, endocarditis, infection, lymphoma, multiple myeloma, nephritis, pregnancy, pulmonary embolism, rheumatoid arthritis, tuberculosis.

**What would cause decreased levels?**

CHF, sickle cell anemia, polycythemia

# Ferritin

**Normal**

20-300 ng/mL

**Indications**

diagnosing iron-deficiency anemia or hemochromatosis, monitor iron levels during pregnancy

**Description**

Ferritin is the storage form of Iron. Some is stored in body tissue, some circulates in the blood. It is formed in the liver spleen and bone marrow. Ferritin in the blood is usually proportional to stored ferritin. Ferritin is a more sensitive and specific test for identifying iron-deficiency anemia, however, it is usually measured in conjunction with total iron binding capacity and iron.

**What would cause increased levels?**

inflammation, breast cancer, hemolytic anemia, fasting, hemochromatosis, liver disease, hyperthyroidism, alcoholism, Hodgkin's disease, infection, leukemia

**What would cause decreased levels?**

dialysis, iron-deficiency anemia

# Folic Acid

## Normal

2 - 20 ng/mL

## Indications

diagnosis of megaloblastic anemia, monitor effects of long-term total parenteral nutrition, identify folate deficiency

## Description

Folate is an essential water soluble vitamin. It is stored in the liver and is an important part of RBC and WBC function, DNA replication, and cell division.

## What would cause increased levels?

Vitamin B12 deficiency, excess folate intake, pernicious anemia

## What would cause decreased levels?

malnutrition, hemolytic anemias, scurvy, liver disease, Crohn's disease, megaloblastic anemia, neoplasm, alcoholism, pregnancy, sideroblastic anemias, ulcerative colitis, whipple's disease.

# Glomerular Filtration Rate

## Normal

60 mL/min/1.73 m2

## Indications

indicator of kidney disease, useful tool in evaluating the extent of kidney damage.

## Description

Glomerular filtration rate (GFR) is an estimate of blood flow through the kidneys. There are different equations used to estimate the GFR. A GFR <60 ml mL/min/1.73 m2 for over 3 months indicates chronic kidney disease. A GFR < 15 mL/min/1.73 m2 indicates kidney failure.

## What would cause increased levels?

N/A

## What would cause decreased levels?

kidney disease, kidney failure

# Glucose

**Normal**

70-115 mg/dL

**Indications**

diagnosis of insulinemia, identifying hypoglycemia, assist in diagnosing diabetes, monitor treatments for diabetes

**Description**

Glucose is a sugar molecule that is a component of carbohydrates. In the body sugar is stored as glycogen in liver and muscle. Glucose is a very important source of energy in the body. The pancreas helps regulate levels of glucose in the blood so that levels are never too high or too low. Glucose levels naturally rise after meals with the intake of carbohydrates.

**What would cause increased levels?**

stress (physical and emotional), pancreatitis, stroke, Cushing's syndrome, DM, hemochromatosis, liver disease, myocardial infarction, pancreatic adenoma, renal disease, shock, trauma, strenuous exercise, Vitamin B1 deficiency

**What would cause decreased levels?**

malabsorption syndromes, alcohol ingestion, glucagon deficiency, von Gierke disease, hypothyroidism, Addison's disease, maple syrup urine disease, starvation, post-gastrectomy,

# Glucose Tolerance Test

### Normal

Fasting: 60-100 mg/dL
1 hour: <200 mg/dL
2 hours: < 140 mg/dL

### Indications

identify impaired glucose metabolism

### Description

The glucose tolerance test (GTT) is a measure of glucose metabolism after a specific amount of glucose intake.  A fasting blood sugar is taken and then a 75 gram carbohydrate drink is taken.  Blood sugars are measured 1 hour, 2 hour, and 3 hour post-prandial.   Blood sugars over 126 mg/dL fasting or >200 mg/dL after 2 hours indicate a problem in glucose metabolism.

### What would cause increased levels?

elevated numbers indicate impaired glucose metabolism

### What would cause decreased levels?

N/A

# Glycosylated Hemoglobin

## Normal

5.6-7.5 % of total hgb

## Indications

assess control of blood sugars over a several month time frame

## Description

Glycosylated hemoglobin (Hgb A1c) is the combination of sugar in the blood (glucose) and hemoglobin. When glucose is elevated in the blood the amount of glycosylated hemoglobin increases proportionally. A red blood cells lifespan is about 4 months, so you can get an idea of blood sugar control over the last several months.

## What would cause increased levels?

DM

## What would cause decreased levels?

renal failure, blood loss, pregnancy, hemolytic anemia.

# Growth Hormone

**Normal**

Male: <5 ng/mL
Female: < 10 ng/mL

**Indications**

diagnosing acromegaly, dwarfism, or gigantism.

**Description**

Growth hormone is secreted by the anterior pituitary. Growth hormone helps regulate sleep and growth throughout childhood. Growth hormone stimulates protein production and lipid and glucose metabolism.

**What would cause increased levels?**

cirrhosis, acromegaly, Exercise, hyperpituitarism, gigantism, malnutrition, anorexia nervosa, diabetes, renal failure, stress

**What would cause decreased levels?**

dwarfism, hypopituitarism

# Hematocrit

### Normal

Male: 41 - 50%
Female: 36 - 44%

### Indications

identify anemia, bleeding, bleeding disorder, fluid imbalances.

### Description

Hematocrit is the percentage of the blood that is made up of packed red blood cells. A hematocrit level of 40% indicates that there are 40 mL packed red blood cells in 100mL of blood.

### What would cause increased levels?

erythrocytosis, polycythemia, shock, dehydration

### What would cause decreased levels?

anemia, blood loss, bone marrow hyperplasia, severe burns,

# Hemoglobin

### Normal

Male: 13.5 - 16.5 g/dL
Female: 12.0 - 15.0 g/dL

### Indications

identify bleeding disorders, anemia, blood loss,

### Description

Hemoglobin is the main protein in red blood cells. It binds to and transports oxygen in the blood, and can also carry carbon dioxide. Hemoglobin is an iron containing compound, And iron-deficiency can affect hemoglobin's ability to carry oxygen.

### What would cause increased levels?

burns, COPD, CHF, dehydration, eryhrocytosis, high altitudes, polycythemia vera

### What would cause decreased levels?

hemolytic disorders, nutrition deficiency, fluid retention, anemias, Hodgkin's disease, hemorrhage, leukemia, carcinoma, lymphoma, pregnancy

# High Density Lipoprotein

### Normal

<60 optimal mg/dL

### Indications

HDL cholesterol is beneficial, and lower levels indicate increased risk for heart disease.

### Description

Cholesterol is transported via lipoproteins. There are multiple types of lipoproteins and they each have slightly different functions: high-density lipoprotein (HDL), low-density lipoprotein, LDL, very low-density lipoprotein (VLDL). HDL cholesterol is considered the good cholesterol as it travels through the blood picking up extra cholesterol and taking it back to the liver.

### What would cause increased levels?

exercise, mono- and poly- unsaturated fats

### What would cause decreased levels?

smoking, high saturated and trans fat diet, excess body weight

# Homocysteine

## Normal

0.54 - 2.3 mg/L

## Indications

identify enzyme deficiencies that cause homocystinuria, evaluate risk of cardiovascular disease or venous thrombosis.

## Description

Homocysteine is an amino acid in the body that can be synthesized from the amino acid methionine. Homocysteine required vitamin B12 and Folate to break it down. Excess homocysteine can damage blood vessels, impact clotting, and increase risk of plaque formation.

## What would cause increased levels?

chronic renal failure, folic acid deficiency, homocystinuria, Vitamin B12 deficiency, coronary artery disease.

## What would cause decreased levels?

N/A

# International Normalized Ratio

## Normal

0.8 - 1.2

## Indications

evaluate therapeutic doses of anticoagulants, identify patients at higher risk for bleeding, identify cause of bleeding, and deficiencies

## Description

International normalized ratio (INR) takes results from a prothrombin time test and standardizes it regardless of collection method.

## What would cause increased levels?

disseminated intravascular coagulation, hereditary factors, liver disease, vitamin k deficiency, SLE, drug therapy,

## What would cause decreased levels?

enteritis, ovarian hyperfunction

# Iron

**Normal**

50-175 ug/dL

**Indications**

identify blood loss, hemochromatosis, malabsorption of iron, iron overload, type of anemia, thalassemia, or sideroblastic anemia

**Description**

Iron is an element that is an important component of hemoglobin in red blood cells. Hemoglobin transports oxygen from the lungs to all the cells of the body. Most of the iron in the body is in hemoglobin, but some iron is in myoglobin and some is stored in the liver, bone marrow, and spleen. The storage form of iron is ferritin. Iron is transported in the blood by a protein called transferrin.

**What would cause increased levels?**

hemolytic anemia, iron poisoning, sideroblastic anemia, acute leukemia, Vitamin B6 deficiency  acute liver disease, hemochromatosis, aplastic anemia, nephritis, thalassemia, pernicious anemia, lead toxicity

**What would cause decreased levels?**

infection, carcinoma, blood loss, hypothyroidism, iron-deficiency anemia, nephrosis, protein malnutrition

# Lactic Acid

## Normal

0.3 -2.6 mMol/L

## Indications

determine cause of acidosis, evaluate tissue oxygenation

## Description

Lactate is a byproduct of carbohydrate metabolism. Lactate is broken down by the liver. During intense exercise pyruvate is converted to lactate to provide a little extra energy when there is not enough oxygen present. If the liver doesn't properly breakdown lactate that can lead to increased levels.

## What would cause increased levels?

DM, heart failure, hemorrhage, excess alcohol consumption, lactic acidosis, pulmonary embolism, reye's syndrome, shock, strenuous exercise.

## What would cause decreased levels?

N/A

# Lipase

## Normal

23 - 300 U/L

## Indications

diagnose pancreatitis, diagnose pancreatic cancer

## Description

Lipase is an enzyme created in the pancreas. It travels to the intestines where it aids in the breakdown of fats. If damage occurs to certain parts of the pancreas lipase is released into the bloodstream.

## What would cause increased levels?

cholecystitis, pancreatic duct obstruction, pancreatic cyst, pseudocyst, pancreatic inflammation, pancreatitis, renal failure.

## What would cause decreased levels?

N/A

# Low Density Lipoprotein

### Normal

<70 mg/dL

### Indications

Useful in determining risk of cardiovascular disease.

### Description

Cholesterol is transported via lipoproteins. There are multiple types of lipoproteins and they each have slightly different functions: high-density lipoprotein (HDL), low-density lipoprotein, LDL, very low-density lipoprotein (VLDL).

### What would cause increased levels?

diet high in saturated fats

### What would cause decreased levels?

regular physical activity

# Magnesium

## Normal

1.6 – 2.6 mg/dL

## Indications

monitor renal failure, chronic alcoholism, monitor cardiac arrhythmias,

## Description

Magnesium is a cation necessary for protein synthesis, nucleic acid synthesis, muscle contraction, ADP (adenosine diphosphate) use, nerve impulse conduction, and blood clotting. Magnesium affects the absorption of sodium, calcium, phosphorus, potassium.

## What would cause increased levels?

Addison's disease, adrenocorticol insufficiency, dehydration, diabetic acidosis, hypothyroidism, SLE, multiple myeloma, overuse of antacids, renal insufficiency, tissue trauma

## What would cause decreased levels?

alcoholism, diabetic acidosis, glomerulonephritis, hemodialysis, hypercalcemia, hypoparathyroidism, inadequate Mg intake, malabsorption, pancreatitis, pregnancy, diarrhea

# Mean corpuscular volume

## Normal

80-100 fl

## Indications

assist in anemia diagnosis, identify hematologic disorders

## Description

Mean corpuscular volume (MCV) is the average of the volume of red blood cells. It is helpful in differentiating between different types of anemia.

## What would cause increased levels?

alcoholism, antimetabolite therapy, liver disease, pernicious anemia, Vitamin B12 anemia, folate anemia

## What would cause decreased levels?

iron-deficiency anemia, thalassemia

# Myoglobin

**Normal**

5-70 ng/mL

**Indications**

identifying damage from a MI or skeletal muscle damage.

**Description**

Myoglobin is a protein in skeletal and cardiac muscle that binds oxygen. When damage is done to heart and skeletal muscle, myoglobin is released into the blood.

**What would cause increased levels?**

rhabdomyolysis, heart surgery, exercise, cocaine use, MI, muscular dystrophy, shock, renal failure

**What would cause decreased levels?**

myasthenia gravis, rheumatoid arthritis

# Osmolality

**Normal**

261 – 280  mOsm/kg

**Indications**

monitor electrolyte balance and acid-base balance, monitor hydration, evaluate function of antidiuretic hormone.

**Description**

Osmolality is a measure of the particles in solution.  The size, shape, and charge of the particles do not impact the osmolality

**What would cause increased levels?**

dehydration, azotemia, hypercalcemia, diabetic ketoacidosis, hypernatremia, diabetes insipidus

**What would cause decreased levels?**

adrenocorticoid insufficiency, hyponatremia, syndrome of inappropriate antidiuretic hormone

# Oxygen Saturation SaO2

**Normal**

95 - 100%

**Indications**

as part of the ABG to determine respiratory status

**Description**

Oxygen is transported in the blood in two ways. Oxygen dissolved in blood plasma (pO2) and oxygen bound to hemoglobin (SaO2). About 97% of oxygen is bound to hemoglobin while 3% is dissolved in plasma. There is a relationship between saturation and partial pressure referred to the oxyhemoglobin dissociation curve. SaO2 of about 90% is associated with PO2 of about 60 mmHg.

# Partial Pressure of CO2

### Normal

35 - 45 mmHg

### Indications

part of the ABG reflects the amount of $CO_2$ dissolved in the blood

### Description

$pCO_2$ is an indirect measure of gas exchange within the lungs.

### What would cause increased levels?

$CO_2$ retention: pulmonary edema, COPD

### What would cause decreased levels?

hyperventilation, hypoxia, anxiety, pregnancy, pulmonary embolism

# Partial Pressure of O2

**Normal**

80 - 100 mmHg

**Indications**

part of an ABG to determine respiratory status

**Description**

Oxygen is transported in the blood in two ways. Oxygen dissolved in blood plasma (pO2) and oxygen bound to hemoglobin (SaO2). About 97% of oxygen is bound to hemoglobin while 3% is dissolved in plasma. There is a relationship between saturation and partial pressure referred to the oxyhemoglobin dissociation curve. SaO2 of about 90% is associated with PO2 of about 60 mmHg

**What would cause increased levels?**

↑ O2 in inhaled air, polycythemia

**What would cause decreased levels?**

↓O2 in inhaled air, anemia, cardiac decompensation, COPD, restrictive pulmonary disease, hypoventilation

# Partial Thromboplastin Time

## Normal

25 - 35 seconds

## Indications

detection of coagulation disorders, evaluate response to anticoagulation medication, preoperative assessment

## Description

Partial Thromboplastin Time (PTT) evaluates the function of factors XII, XI, IX, VII, V, X, II, and I, represents the amount of time required for a fibrin clot to form

## What would cause increased levels?

DIC, factor deficiencies, liver disease, vitamin K deficiency, polycythemia, dialysis, Von Willebrand's disease

## What would cause decreased levels?

N/A

# pH (partial pressure of Hydrogen ion)

## Normal

7.35 - 7.45

## Description

reflects the amount of free H+ ions in the body

## What would cause increased levels?

Metabolic alkalosis - suctioning, potassium depletion, diarrhea, vomiting

Respiratory alkalosis - stimulation of the respiratory center, hyperventilation, fever

## What would cause decreased levels?

Metabolic acidosis- DKA, decreased excretion of H+, increased acid intake

Respiratory acidosis - asthma, bronchoconstriction, emphysema, pneumonia

# Phosphorus

**Normal**

3.0-4.5 mg/dL

**Indications**

diagnosing hyperparathyroidism, evaluation of renal failure

**Description**

Phosphorus is a major intracellular anion playing a vital role in cellular metabolism.  it makes up the phospholipid bilayer of the cell membrane, and is crucial in the formation of bones and teeth. Calcium and phosphorus share an inverse relationship

**What would cause increased levels?**

excess vitamin D, DKA, lactic acidosis, renal failure (excreted by kidneys), pulmonary embolism, respiratory acidosis, hypocalcemia, acromegaly

**What would cause decreased levels?**

hyperalimentation, hyperinsulinism, hyperparathyroidism, hypokalemia, hypercalcemia, alkalosis, vomiting and diarrhea, malnutrition, osteomalacia

# Platelets

## Normal

100,000 - 450,000 cells/mcL

## Indications

determine clotting vs bleeding disorders, part of a basic screening exam

## Description

platelets play a role in coagulation, hemostasis, and thrombus formation.  Platelets are the smallest blood cell, damaged vessels send out signals that result in platelets traveling to the area and becoming "active".

## What would cause increased levels?

infection, bone marrow disorders (polycythemia vera), RA, malignancy, cirrhosis, pancreatitis, trauma

## What would cause decreased levels?

aplastic anemia, alcoholism, medication, inherited, carcinoma, lymphoma, uremia, hemorrhage, DIC, bacterial infection, Idiopathic thrombocytopenic purpura, radiation, dialysis

# Potassium

**Normal**

3.5 - 5.5 mEq/L

**Indications**

evaluate electrolyte imbalances, useful in evaluating cardiac arrhythmias, useful when patient is receiving diuretic therapy, useful with acidotic patients

**Description**

potassium is the most abundant intracellular cation and plays a vital role in the transmission of electrical impulses in cardiac and skeletal muscle. It plays a role in acid base equilibrium. In states of acidosis hydrogen with enter the cell as this happens it will force potassium out of the cell, a 0.1 decrease in pH will cause a 0.5 increase in K+.

**What would cause increased levels?**

acidosis, renal failure, diet, dialysis, burns, Addison's disease, ketoacidosis, trauma, hyperventilation, uremia

**What would cause decreased levels?**

CHF, alkalosis, hyperaldosteronism, toxic shock syndrome, malabsorption, excess insulin, Cushing's

# Prealbumin

**Normal**

19-38 mg/dL

**Indications**

helpful in evaluating nutritional status

**Description**

protein produced by the liver, short half-life (2 days) making it a good indicator of protein status and malnutrition

**What would cause increased levels?**

steroid therapy, alcoholism

**What would cause decreased levels?**

malnutrition, chronic illness, inflammatory process, trauma, liver disease

# Prostate Specific Antigen

### Normal

Male: < 4 ng/mL
Female: < 0.5 ng/mL

### Indications

utilized to evaluate enlarged prostate when prostate cancer is suspected, stage cancer, evaluate effectiveness of treatments

### Description

PSA produced by prostate when used in conjunction with digital exam this test is helpful in diagnosing and assessing prostate abnormalities

### What would cause increased levels?

BPH, prostate cancer, urinary retention

### What would cause decreased levels?

N/A

# Protein (total)

### Normal

6 - 8 g/dL

### Indications

diagnosing myeloma, lymphoma, macroglobulinemia, amyloidosis, evaluate kidney function

### Description

Protein is an important contributor of energy in our diet. Protein has many numerous functions in the body

### What would cause increased levels?

UTI, nephrotic syndrome, heavy metal poisoning, exercise, diabetic nephropathy, multiple myeloma, sickle cell disease, sarcoidosis, lymphoproliferative disorder

### What would cause decreased levels?

N/A

# Prothrombin Time

## Normal

11 - 14 seconds

## Indications

evaluate therapeutic doses of anticoagulants, identify patients at higher risk for bleeding, identify cause of bleeding, and deficiencies

## Description

time it takes for a fibrin clot to form.  Prothrombin is produced by the liver and is dependent on vitamin K.

## What would cause increased levels?

disseminated intravascular coagulation, hereditary factors, liver disease, vitamin k deficiency, SLE, drug therapy,

## What would cause decreased levels?

enteritis, ovarian hyperfunction

# Red Blood Cell

## Normal

Male:  4.5 - 5.5 x10$^6$/cells/mm$^3$
Female: 4.0 - 4.9 x10$^6$/cells/mm$^3$

## Indications

helpful in identifying anemia, determine blood loss, part of the CBC and useful in a general physical exam.

## Description

Red blood cells (RBCs) contain hemoglobin which is responsible for oxygen transport throughout the body.  RBCs are primarily produced in the bone marrow, they have a life span of 120 days and are destroyed in the spleen and liver. RBC production is regulated by erythropoietin which is produced and released from the kidneys.

## What would cause increased levels?

dehydration, polycythemia vera, COPD, bone marrow failure

## What would cause decreased levels?

chemotherapy, anemia, hemorrhage, leukemia, organ failure, hypervolemia, pregnancy

# Red Blood Cell Distribution Width

**Normal**

<14.5

**Indications**

Useful in the diagnosis of anemia

**Description**

Red blood cell distribution width (RDW) is a measurement of the variation of RBC cell size amongst the entire population of RBCs. Used with other red cell indices to determine cause of anemia.

**What would cause increased levels?**

Anemia, when combined with additional RBC indices specific cause for anemia can be better determined

**What would cause decreased levels?**

N/A

# Sodium (serum)

**Normal**

135-145 mEq/L

**Indications**

the sodium ion is mostly found in the serum (extracellular) the test helps to evaluate total body sodium stores

**Description**

Sodium (Na) is the most abundant cation in extracellular fluid. Sodium aids in osmotic pressure, renal retention and excretion of water, acid-base balance, regulation of other cations and anions in the body, plays a role in blood pressure regulation, and stimulation of neuromuscular reactions. Generally speaking elevated sodium levels are often due to relative deficit of free water.

**What would cause increased levels?**

Cushing's disease, dehydration, burn injury, azotemia (elevated nitrogen), vomiting, lactic acidosis, fever, excessive iv fluids containing saline, diarrhea, diabetes,

**What would cause decreased levels?**

CHF, cystic fibrosis, diuretic use, metabolic acidosis, Addison's disease, nephrotic syndrome, excessive ADH, liver failure

# Triglycerides

**Normal**

<150 mg/dL

**Indications**

evaluate for elevated triglycerides, estimate risk for atherosclerotic heart disease and stroke

**Description**

triglycerides are required to provide energy during the metabolic process, excess triglycerides are stored in adipose tissue

**What would cause increased levels?**

MI, alcoholism, anorexia nervosa, cirrhosis, HTN, nephrotic syndrome, obesity, renal failure, pancreatitis, stress

**What would cause decreased levels?**

COPD, liver disease, hyperthyroidism, malnutrition, malabsorption

# Total Iron Binding Capacity

**Normal**

250-460 ug/dL

**Indications**

assess cause of anemia and whether anemia is associated with iron deficiency or another cause, assess iron metabolism and storage

**Description**

Total iron binding capacity is essentially a measure to determine if a patient has too much or too little iron in the body and how well iron is being transported

**What would cause increased levels?**

liver disease, iron-deficiency anemia, pregnancy

**What would cause decreased levels?**

infection, cirrhosis, protein depletion, renal disease

# Troponin I

### Normal

*There is a wide range of normal values among varying institutions and texts with regard to Troponin I. It is essential to verify institutional norms.*

< 0.035 ng/mL

### Indications

evaluating damage to heart muscle, diagnose an MI

### Description

Troponins are proteins that initiate contraction of muscle fibers. Troponin I is specific to heart muscle. Troponins stays elevated for a week after muscle damage then returns to normal.

### What would cause increased levels?

heart damage, MI

### What would cause decreased levels?

N/A

# White Blood Cell

## Normal

4,500 - 10,000 cells/mcL

## Indications

white blood cells demonstrate the body's response or ability to respond to an infectious process

## Description

White blood cells are created in the bone marrow, their primary function is to defend the body against infection.   There are various types of WBCs which have different shapes and functions.

## What would cause increased levels?

(leukocytosis) pregnancy, emotional stress, transfusion reaction, infection, Cushing's disease, leukemia (unnatural rise in immature WBCs)

## What would cause decreased levels?

radiation, SLE, anemia, rheumatoid arthritis, viral infection

# Get a FREE PDF download of the Lab Charts at NRSNG.com/Labs

# Thank You!

Before you go, I'd like to sincerely say "Thank You" for purchasing this book.

I know you could have picked dozens of laboratory books and I am thrilled that you chose this one. I am confident that it will help you with your studies.

I'd like to ask you for a small ***FAVOR***. <u>Could you please take a minute to leave a review for this book on AMAZON.</u>

This feedback will help me to continue to write books that help you in your nursing studies. The review will also help others to find this book. If you loved the book, please let me know ; - ).

Happy Nursing!

-Jon Haws RN BSN

## More Kindle Books by Jon Haws and NRSNG.com

<u>Essential EKG: EKG Interpretation, Rhythms, Arrhythmia</u>
<u>Human Body: Human Anatomy for Kids an Inside Look at Body Organs</u>

Made in the USA
Lexington, KY
05 November 2015